Introduction.

I have writen this simple guide to weight loss and weight management to help get you on your way to a healthier, happier you. Burn Fat Fast is an easy to follow guide which gives you the important information you need to give you a jump start to a vibrant, radiant and sexy new you!

If you are tired of counting calories, fat grams and points and you are tired of diets that just do not work, then this book is for you.

I don't even like to call this a "weight loss" book as it's so much more than that. It is a total nutrition book with the"side effect" of weight loss! So how would you like that for a side effect?

As a person who has battled the bulge myself I understand that it is possible for people to be overweight by no "real" fault of their own. Why? Well beause there is a lot of misleading information out there on this subject and a lot of so-called quick fixes from fad diets to misleading advice. The reality is that even though it may not seem so at the time the easiest way for most people to loose weight is to change their habits with regards to food and exercising.

The purpose of this book is to provide you with the information you need to make the right choices for you, so you can take steps to lower your weight and maintain a healthy weight.

Table of Contents

Foreword

Losing weight can't be achieved in just a wink of an eye. Before you reach your main goal, you have to do accurate steps and get rid of your unhealthy lifestyle. Depending on your preferred schemes, losing weight can complicated or easy.

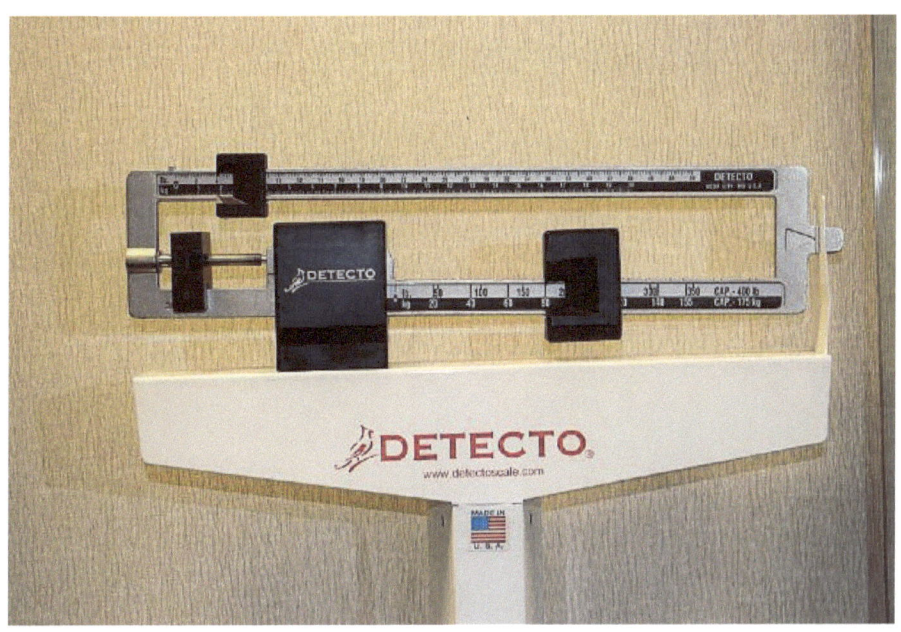

Chapter 1:

Introduction

<u>Synopsis</u>

Weight loss requires a reduction in calorie consumption. Most people try to reduce weight through exercising or dieting.

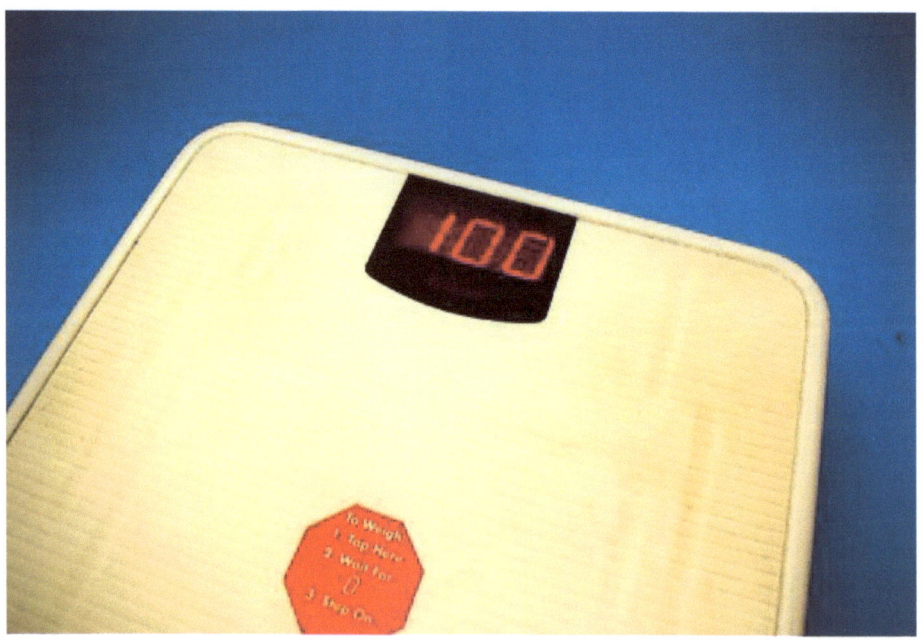

Basic Information

Every person has their own reason why they opt to lose weight. Some of them desire to develop their self-confidence or appear more attractive while others just want to stay healthy and fit. Whatever reasons you have, there is nothing to worry about. Achieving a perfect body and weight can be done without practising any complicated procedures. It is a matter of how you control and motivate yourself to live a healthy lifestyle.

To know more about weight loss and maintenance, this book will serve you as an ultimate guide. Through this, you have a chance to recognize its fundamental facts. So, start reading this book and start improving your weight condition and lifestyle.

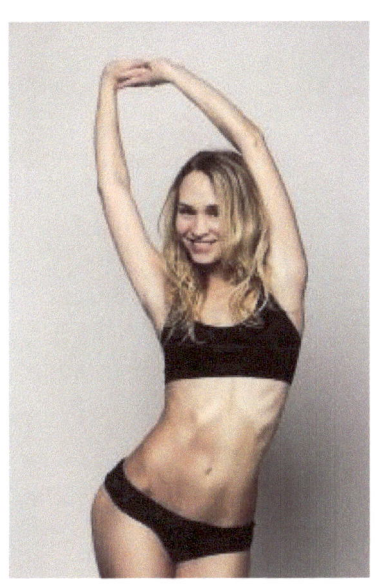

Chapter 2:

Weight Loss – Its Definition and Types

<u>Synopsis</u>

Whether you want to stay fit, switch your body into a perfect one or appear sexier, you have to understand the entire concept of weight loss. If you regularly read health news, you probably recognize that the rate of obesity tends to increase. This alarming condition has awakened health practitioners and organizations. As a result, they are providing adequate tips and solutions to solve this issue. However, the help of these health agencies is not enough.

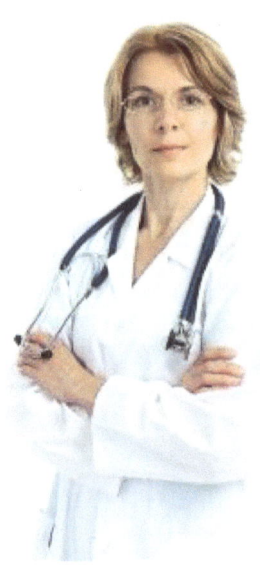

Weight Loss Definition and Types

If you really want to reduce your weight, you have to help yourself. You have to be more conscious with your daily lifestyle and activities.

Weight loss refers to a reduction of the total body mass characterized by a loss of skeletal muscle and body fats. This term comes in two types:

• Intentional Weight Loss – When a person intentionally reduces weight, they often plan a dietary or training program. These programs are designed to lose a certain amount of weight within a short period of time.

• Unintentional Weight Loss - Weight loss may be accidental if a person is suffering from any untreated health issues. The typical examples of these are diabetes, stress, anxiety and a lot more.

As experts claim, losing weight offers multiple benefits. Aside from a stunning appearance, you also have a chance to live for more years. Obese people often suffer from multiple diseases such as diabetes, hypertension, heart disease and cancer.

Weight Management Defined

Weight management is defined as an enduring approach to a healthy lifestyle. It covers a balance of physical exercise and healthy eating to link energy intake and energy expenditure.

Understanding the needs of your body is essential to weight management.

It can also control over and under consumption of foods. Nutritionists claim that weight management does not cover fad diets.

It often focuses on the long-term outcomes followed by body weight maintenance. If you manage your weight, you can achieve not only a perfect figure, but prevent chronic diseases as well.

Methods of Weight Management.

Weight management comes in multiple methods. Some are easy to follow while others need constant monitoring and strict implementation. To get more details about these schemes, here are some of its various methods you should know.

Weight Loss Considerations and Tips .

Even if you opt to shed extra pounds instantly, it is still essential to avoid crash diets, fad diets, frequent fasting and other intense weight loss measures.

These schemes can put you at risk for health problems.

Say for instance, people who use laxatives while dieting may develop dehydration, kidney problems, heart issues and intestinal damage.

The best way to lose more weight is to make a diet that covers adequate healthy foods. This can help in maintaining body function while shedding pounds of weight. Before doing any activities or engaging with any program, make sure that you consult with your nutritionist or doctor.

While making a weight loss plan, you should always include proper exercise. Aside from burning calories through intense physical activity, regular training develops a resting metabolism. Therefore, it can help the body to burn more calories while performing ordinary activities.

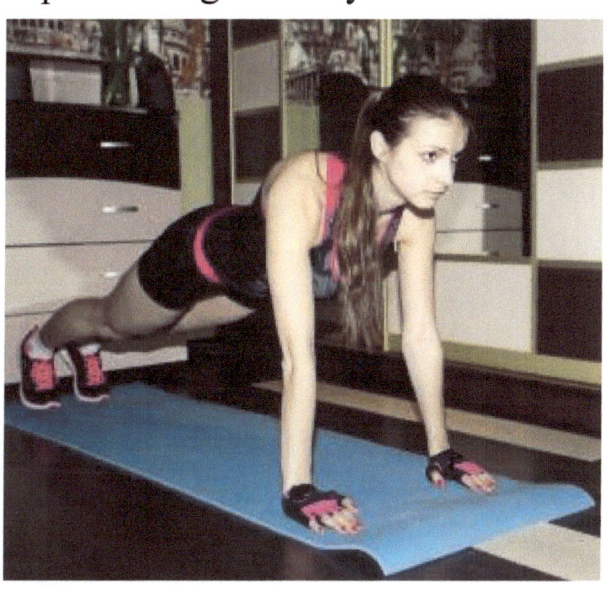

Chapter 3:

What is a healthy diet?

<u>Synopsis</u>

Not all people are aware of how to lose weight. Sometimes, they just depend on several programs that aim to reduce more body fat and achieve a perfect figure. Before you start reducing your fat, you should understand first the fundamental fact of weight management.

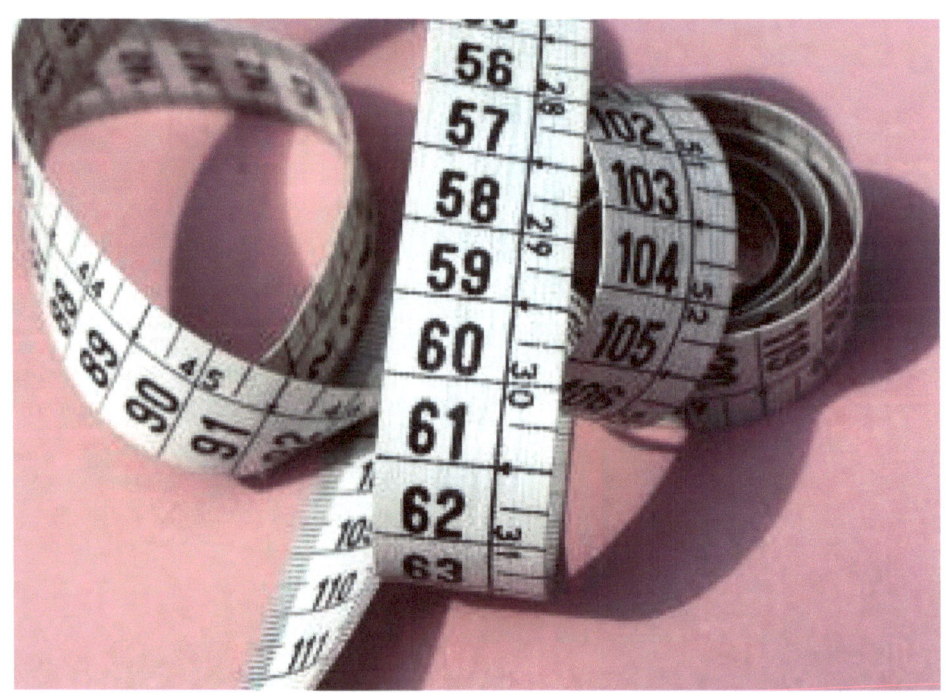

What do I eat?

Do you eat only when you are hungry? Or do you simply eat when you can? Eating the right foods and in the right proportion is of extreme importance.

A healthy diet is one that helps to maintain and improve your health. It assists in the prevention of chronic diseases such as cancer, diabetes, heart attack and the list goes on. How do you know the right proportion to eat at any given time? As you continue to read this book, I will guide you through the steps you need to take on your quest to a new affordable healthy way of life.

A healthy diet consists of a variety of fruits, vegetables, whole grains, includes lean meats, poultry, fish, beans and nuts and is low in saturated and Trans fats, cholesterol, salt (sodium) and sugars and stays within your daily calorie needs.

The best way to get all the vitamins, minerals and nutrients your body needs is to eat a variation of foods. No one food or supplement for that matter can provide your body with all you need to keep healthy on a daily basis. Now that we have identified what a healthy diet consists of let's get right into managing the proportions we eat. The next chapter in this book will give you a step by step guide on your daily food intake and how important it is for LIFE!

Eating the right proportions

Having established that your body needs a well-balanced diet with a good supply of vitamins, minerals, a certain amount of protein, carbohydrates – especially high fibre foods, you now need to know how to fit this in your everyday routine. Take a close look at the following guideline.

Eat three meals per day:

This is normally made up of breakfast, a smaller snack or lunch type meal and one main meal. You may decide however, that you need a small snack during the course of the day. Make this a piece of fruit or some nuts.

Meals should be based on a serving of carbohydrate, such as whole meal bread, pasta, wholegrain cereals, brown rice and potatoes, along with fruits and vegetables. The main meal should include a source of lean protein, along with carbohydrate and fruits and vegetables.

Lean sources of protein as mentioned above are: Fish, shellfish, poultry and lean red meat. Get into the habit of eating a small amount of fat. Use olive oil, sesame oil or walnut oil for cooking. Please keep the quantity low.

Drink **alkaline** water daily. Alkaline water helps fibre in your food to swell and perform its duties effectively. It also helps to metabolize other nutrients from your food and keep your skin and hair healthy and prevent your body from becoming dehydrated. You will see a separate chapter on alkaline water as you continue to read this book.

Here is a complete meal plan for your three daily meals as mentioned above

BREAKFAST

- Choose a smart cereal – oatmeal for example.
- Serving of 3-4 assorted fruits.
- Two slices of toast with sardines on top.

LUNCH

Your lunch should not be too heavy but sufficient to fill you up!

Choice # 1

- Green salad with tuna or chicken breast, light salad dressing, about 5-6 whole wheat crackers and 6 ounces light yogurt.

Choice # 2

- Turkey wrap (made with whole-wheat tortilla, lettuce, light mayo, tomato and veggies of choice). **This is very filling!** You can still have ½ cup of sugar free pudding.

Keep your lunch beverages healthy as well. Drink an 8oz bottle of alkaline water and/or a small bottle of natural fruit juice.

<u>DINNER</u>

- Oven baked chicken served with vegetables (an assortment of steamed vegetables would be good. Use broccoli, cauliflower, zucchini and bell peppers for instance). Of course you can change this around based in your personal choices.

- You can add one cup of steamed brown rice as well. Have a glass of alkaline water after you have eaten your meal or your choice of fresh fruit juice.

****Important Note****

Please note that you need to wait at least two (2) hours after having dinner to go to bed. This is necessary as it helps in the digestion process and prevents ulcers and heartburn.

Exploring How to Eat Right to Lose Weight

If you wish to lose weight, you need to focus on your daily meals. You have to know not only the foods that you need to eat, but also the foods that can trigger your weight condition. Instead of worrying about this issue, here are some tips you should consider:

• Know the Exact Foods You Need to Consume – Some people restrain themselves from eating to reduce weight. This scheme is not advisable. If you are hungry, then, you need to eat but with limitations. If you keep on eating fewer amounts of food, you might suffer from complicated health problems like fatigue.

• Consume More Fresh Vegetables and Fruits – Nutritious foods can help you lose weight. These foods are perfect instead of consuming unhealthy meals every day. If you switch into a healthy lifestyle, expect that you will lose weight and have a perfect body condition.

• Avoid Skipping Meals – If you keep on skipping meals, you may become hungrier for the next meal. As much as possible, you need to eat five to six times a day. But, you have to eat a small amount. Never multi-task and don't watch television while eating. While eating, just sit and pay attention to your food.

• Drink More Water – Your body needs more water. Drinking more water is highly recommended than consuming soda drinks. Before eating, you have to drink some water to reduce your food intake. This can help in reducing more body fat.

• Make a Journal – Making a journal is an effective way to monitor your daily eating habits. Depending on your preferred meals, you need to jot it down and you will know the exact amount of food you intake.

• Try New Foods – Even if you are planning to lose weight, it doesn't mean that you need to deprive yourself from eating your favourite foods. Instead of eating the same types of food over and over again, you need to try new and healthy recipes.

• Clean Your Kitchen – It means that you need to remove all food that can destroy your regular healthy diet. As much as possible, buy only some food that is suggested by your nutritionist. This is an excellent move to refrain you from eating your favourite chips or other unhealthy foods.

Through your knowledge on how to eat right, you don't have to worry about your weight and body condition. You can easily motivate yourself to reduce more fat. If you are still confused on how to eat right, you are free to consult your nutritionist.

• More Protein Intake – Food specialists claim that protein intake at breakfast has higher effect compared to succeeding meals. It also consists of a greater thermo genic effect than fats and carbohydrates. If you consume high protein food during breakfast, it helps increase the activity of glycogen.

• Use Smaller Plates – Through the use of smaller plates, it helps you to consume smaller portions of foods. Therefore, chances to eat fewer calories are observed. If you keep on using larger plates, you are always tempted to consume greater portions and that leads to weight gain.

• Consume Low Calorie Foods – An average decrease in calorie intake always lead to slow weight loss. Picking lettuce, broccoli, grapefruit, cauliflower and other low calorie foods is highly recommended.

• Eating More Dairy Foods – Most nutritionists claim that consuming dairy foods can reduce body fat. It happens because a greater amount of dietary calcium develops the amount of energy and fat removed from the body.

• Give Up Soda or Sugary Drinks – One of the main contributors in weight gain is sugary drinks. Even if these drinks are delicious and appear harmless, carbonated drinks consist of a large amount of calories. To avoid calories, you should always drink more water.

Experts suggest the consumption of eight to ten glasses of water regularly.

Take note that there is nothing wrong with you eating food. Just make sure that you are eating the right and healthy ones. You also need to monitor your daily intake to avoid weight gain. If you are motivated and committed to your specific goal, you can achieve it no matter what it takes.

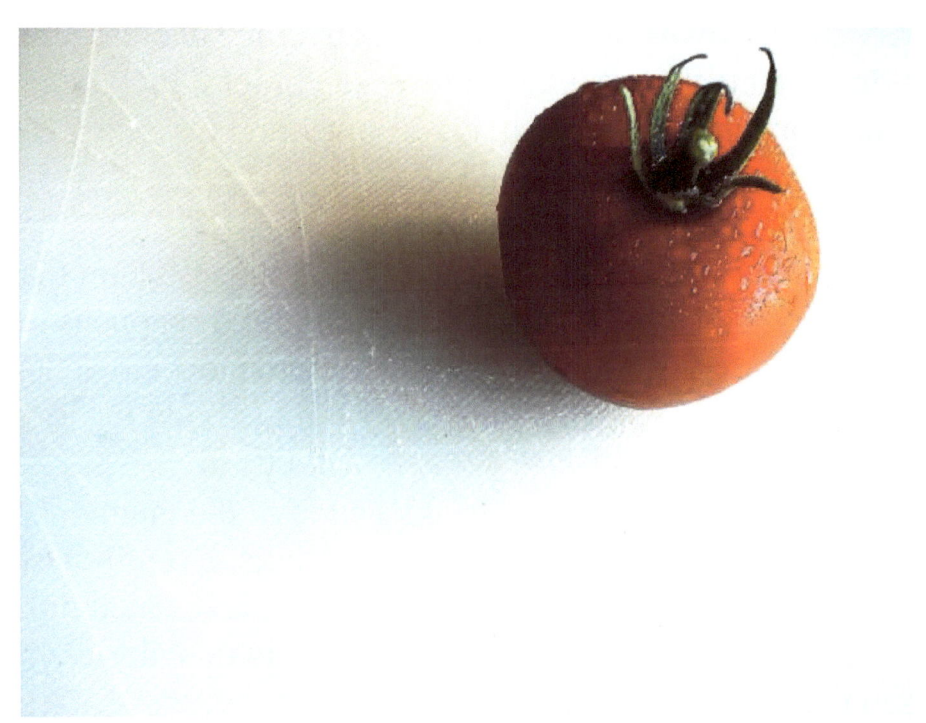

Chapter 4:

Pills and Surgery Basics

<u>Synopsis</u>

To lose weight, some people prefer to purchase supplements or pills. Others also desire to undergo several surgical procedures. Whatever options you will take, you have to be more knowledgeable on how they work.

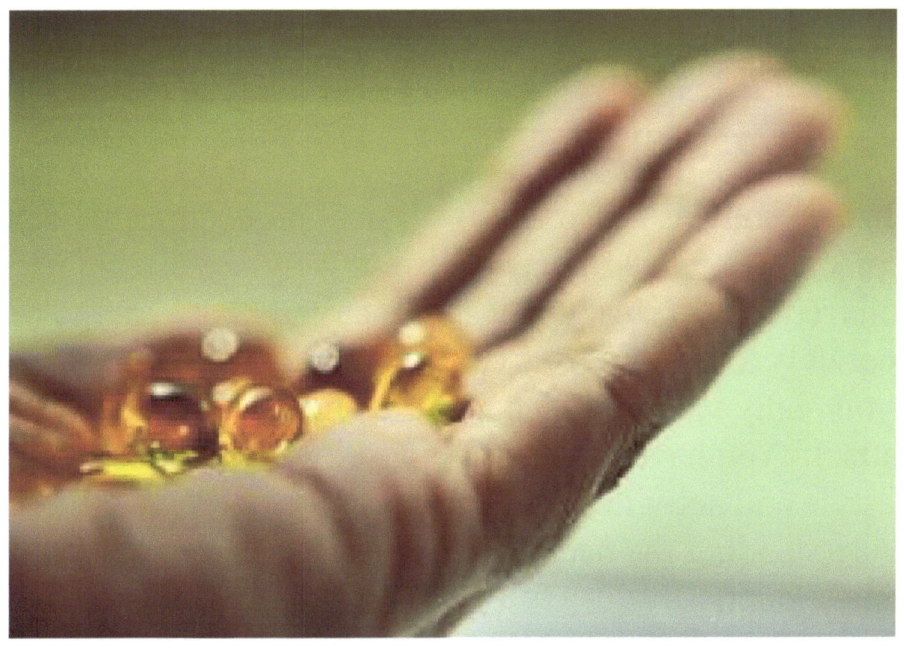

Surgery – How Effective It Is for Losing Weight?

For those who can afford it, they prefer to depend on surgical procedures to remove their excessive body fat. If you are one of them, you have to find the best surgeon. Searching for the best surgeon is not too difficult. You can find one through asking assistance from your trusted friends. You can also read some reviews online to get a reliable surgeon.

Surgical procedures for losing weight are also effective. However, you have to follow the prescriptions of your surgeon before and after the surgery. You also need to be more conscious with your daily activities to avoid any side effects.

Whether you wish to undergo surgical procedures, take pills or practice the natural way of losing weight, you can get your preferred results. Just make sure that you know how to do it accurately to ensure positive outcomes.

If you really want to reduce your weight, you have to help yourself. You have to be more conscious with your daily lifestyle and activities.

Understanding the needs of your body is essential to weight management.

It can also control over and under consumption of foods. Nutritionists claim that weight management does not cover fad diets.
It often focuses on the long-term outcomes
followed by body weight maintenance. If you manage your weight, you can achieve not only a perfect figure, but prevent chronic diseases as well.

Methods of Weight Management.

Weight management comes in multiple methods. Some are easy to follow while others need constant monitoring and strict implementation. To get more details about these schemes, here are some of its various methods you should know.

Chapter 5:

Alkaline Water health benefits

Synopsis

Drinking water is a must every day. It doesn't matter if you do not feel thirsty. You should aim drink some water during the course of the day. See below some important points to consider.

Alkaline Water on the pH scale

Before I elaborate on the health benefits of this amazing water, I want to take a minute to explain alkaline water and the pH scale. Alkaline water is water that is neither acidic nor neutral on the pH scale. It is on the alkaline side of the scale. The pH scale ranges from 0 on the acidic end to 14 on the alkaline end. A solution is neutral if its pH is 7. Substances with a less pH than 7 are acidic while substances with a pH greater than 7 are alkaline. Alkaline water has a pH of approximately 9.5, depending on the brand of the equipment used to alkalize that water. The pH scale is a log scale so a change of one pH unit means a tenfold change in the concentration of hydrogen ions.

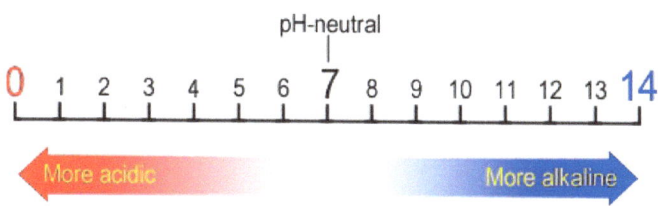

The pH Scale

What does alkaline water do for you?

Keeping yourself alkaline is your first line of defence to fighting any disease. A body that is too acidic provides the ideal environment for diseases to manifest and thrive. One of the primary causes of disease is chronic cellular dehydration, a condition which leaves the body's cells in a perpetual state of weakness and defence. Drinking alkaline water helps this condition and can be up to six times more hydrating than conventional drinking water.

The benefits of alkaline water are immeasurable. This water is essential for consistent and continued health. Let us take a closer look at more health benefits.

Alkaline water:

- Improves your immune system function to help fight diseases.

- Neutralizes the acidity of the body caused by stress, modern diet and air pollution.

- A higher pH in the body reduces the need for fat and cholesterol to protect the body from damaging acids.

- Tastes lighter with a pleasantly sweet flavour.

- Improves the body's absorption of essential nutrients.

- Improves the taste and quality of foods.

- Helps create a greater energy level.

- Improves body functions by cleaning cells from the inside out.

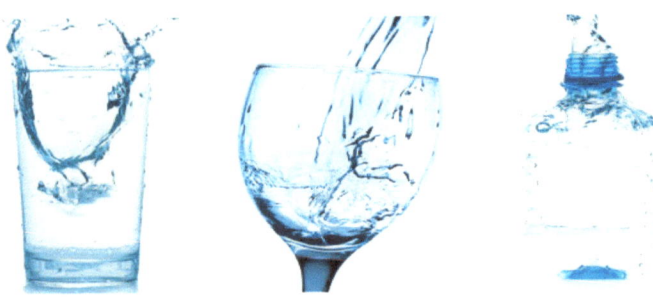

Chapter 6:

Synopsis

Not all people are aware of how to lose weight. Sometimes, they just depend on several programs that aim to reduce more body fat and achieve a perfect figure. Before you start reducing your fat, you should understand first the fundamental facts of weight management.

How to maintain the right body weight

A healthy body weight is a weight range (not any one ideal weight) appropriate for a particular height and body built. A healthy weight should not be confused with a thin weight. Be too thin or constantly trying to get thin with one diet after another is not healthy physically or emotionally. So what is the right body weight? Read on and you will be pleasantly enlightened.

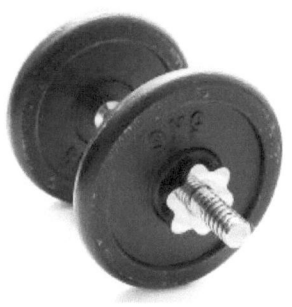

There is no magic pill or hard core exercise program that will help you to get to and maintain that right body weight. Regular physical activity coupled with healthy eating ***not dieting*** promises to be the best way to achieve and maintain the right body weight. Getting physically active does not mean that you have to enrol in a gym and exercise 4-5 times per week. It could be a simple exercise such as walking your dog, riding a bike, dancing or hiking.

What is your BMI (Body Mass Index)?

Ok, so your BMI is the easiest way to determine if you are overweight or underweight. A lot of people think that they are overweight even if they aren't. Just because you do not look like a supermodel does not mean that you are bigger than you should be. In fact, everybody should have some body fat! The average male should expect his body fat to be 10-18 percent of his body weight and the average female should in fact be 18-25 percent of her body weight.

The BMI (body mass index) should be used as a guide and should by no means replace a visit to your health practioner. So here goes.......

This is a breakdown of your BMI based on your weight and height. Please note that your weight is calculated in pounds and not kilograms.

Weight of 120 lbs with a height of 5 feet 6 inches

Your BMI is **19.38**

18-34 years old – Healthy (BMI between 19-24)
35 and older – Healthy (BMI between 19-26)

This shows that this individual is healthy

Weight of 250 lbs with a height of 6 feet

Your BMI is **33.92**

18-34 years old – overweight (BMI over 30)
35 and older – overweight (BMI over 30)

This shows that this individual is overweight (obese)

Healthy BMI would be 18-34 years old – 19-24 or over 35 years old a BMI of
 19-26

You can visit any online resource and calculate your own BMI.

The purpose of calculating your BMI is to ascertain if your weight is in good order and if not you need to do something about it. As you read on in this book you will find that eating the right foods and exercising is the ideal way to keep your weight in check. The absolutely great thing is that you do not have to go on an expensive weight loss program but you are able to choose what you consume and find where you spend the same amount of money on your weekly grocery bill or even less! Isn't that great news???

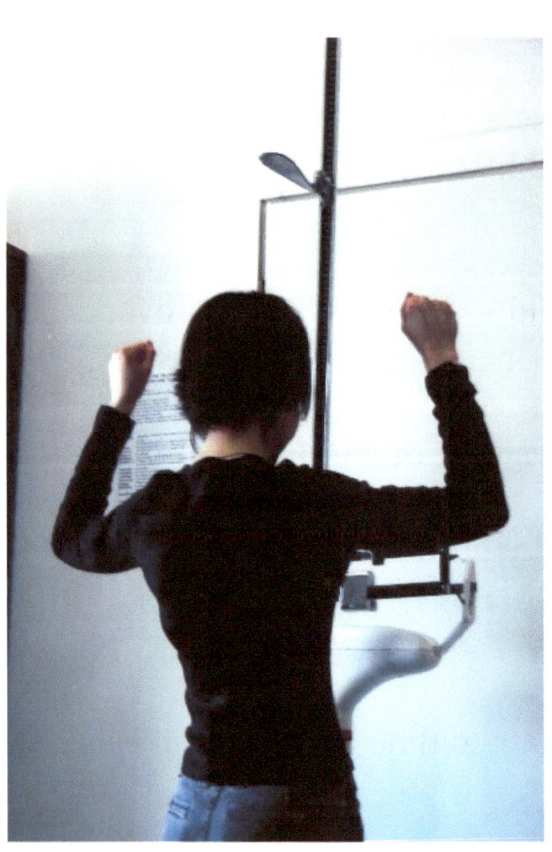

Chapter 7:

Synopsis

The food pyramid basically gives you a visual of what you should be eating every day. The most important thing to consider is proportion. Take a look at the below.

The food pyramid

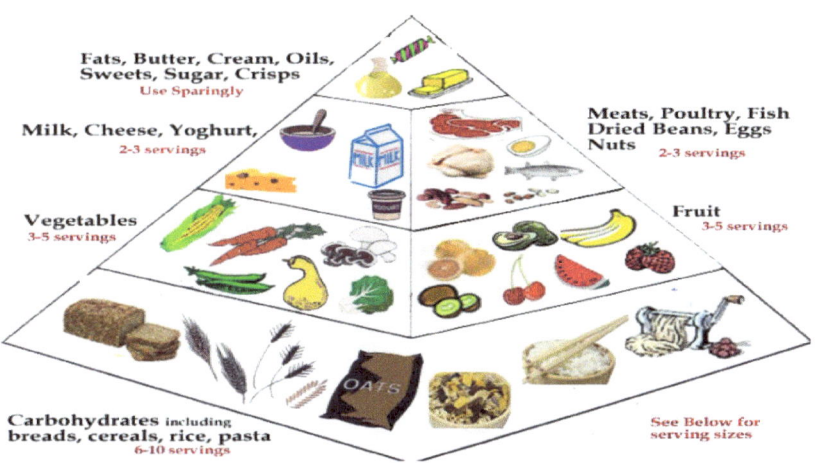

The food/plate proportion

Here is an example of the typical proportions which makes up a complete meal. Please take special note of the fact that this gives you a general idea of the different choices which you have. You need to choose one or two of the items depicted below for your meals with the exception of the veggies and fruits of course which can be 3-5 different choices.

Do you realise the small amount of oils and dairy products which are needed? Special emphasis is placed on fruits and vegetables, whole grains and legumes. Remember wheat is a good source of fibre.

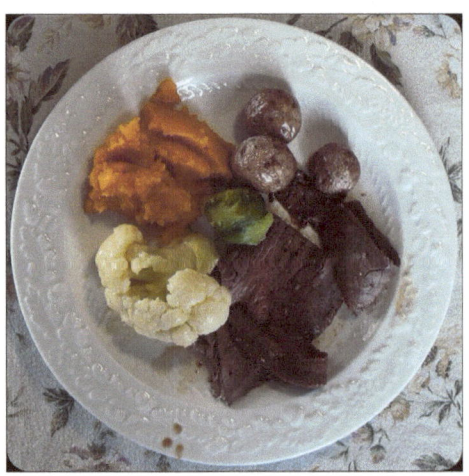

Chapter 8:

Synopsis

People choose to lose weight for various reasons. The benefits can be tremendous if you follow the right routine and manage your diet appropriately.

Significance of Weight Loss Management

If you are not familiar with these benefits, here they are:
• Appear Sexy and Attractive – If you keep on asking why most people prefer to lose weight, most of them give similar answers. Both men and women wish to reduce more body fat to make them sexier.
• Look Healthier and Active – If you are planning to lose weight, you need to eat nutritious foods like fruits and vegetables. As a result, you will achieve a perfect body figure while getting the benefit of practicing a healthy lifestyle.
• Saves More Money – When you are losing weight, you need to consume healthy foods. Therefore, you don't need to buy any food that can destroy your eating habits. This can help you by saving you more cash.
• Know How to handle Your Health Condition – If you wish to lose weight, you should probably start by consulting your doctor. Through this, you will learn several things about how to lose weight and how to live healthy.
With the various benefits of weight loss, everyone is

encouraged to deal with reliable dietary and training programs. Like others, you don't need to rely on multiple programs. Though you keep on entering in several activities, it will never be effective if you don't have self-control or motivation. So, make sure that you always follow your schedule to ensure effective results.

-30-Weight loss management is not too complicated.

Weight loss management is not too complicated. If you have a specific goal, all you need to do is to find ways of how to achieve it. Through the help of weight loss management, you are guided to the specific activities you need to do. You will also know the different foods that you need to eat.

For beginners, they may find it hard to follow their schedules. However, if they are eager to reach their goal, everything will turn out to be fine. This is the reason why most people prefer to lose weight using a special management program.

Are you worried about your excessive fat? If yes, then, you don't need to suffer from its consequences. Don't allow other people to bully you just because your physical appearance. If you are obese, then, you need to find ways to solve this at hand. Through practicing a weight loss plan and management, everything will be in good condition. After several weeks and months, you will realize that you are losing more fat.

Whether you want to lose weight or just want to maintain a healthy body figure, there is always a specific way of how to achieve that goal. After burning more fat, you are confident to face other people. You are also free to wear any apparel you like.

Through following these different guides, you are free to do everything you want. So, start changing your daily activity now! Learn how to practice a healthy lifestyle and see how it affects your weight condition.

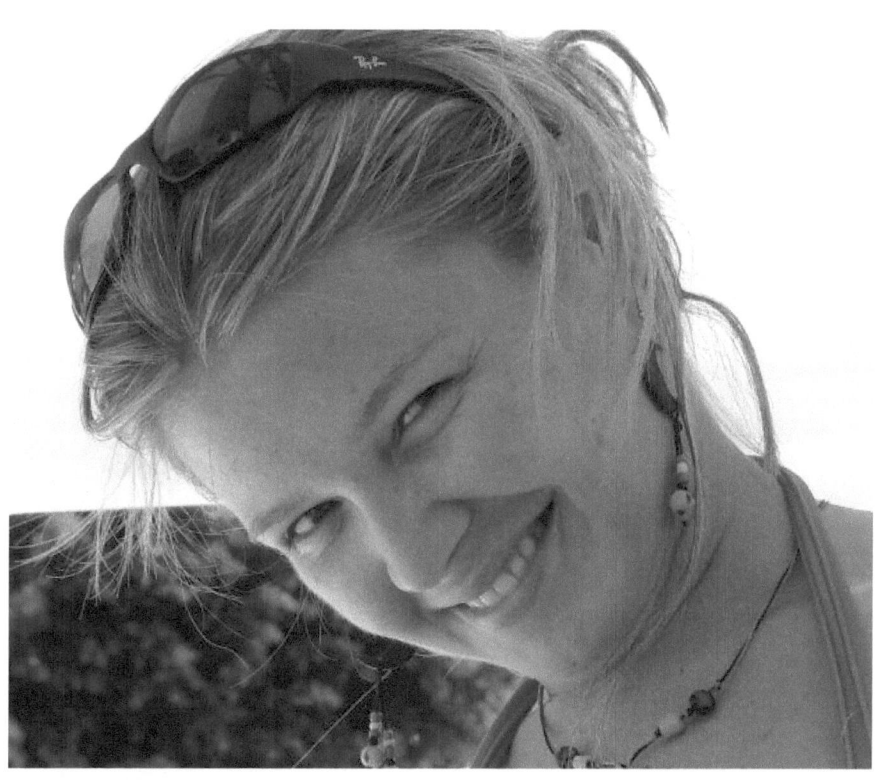

www.ingramcontent.com/pod-product-compliance
Lightning Source LLC
Chambersburg PA
CBHW051128290526
45796CB00001B/6